Essential Oils:
Top 30 Summer And Spring Essential Oil Diffuser Recipes

Table of content

Introduction

Essential oils play a significant role in carrying out our routine activities without any hurdle and without facing any kind of ambiguity. As you know that these oils are just the extracts of different kinds of herbs and are used for fulfilling many kinds of purposes.

The essence of these herbs and plants is very useful in a way that in case you opt for dried herbs for any purpose, a huge quantity of them is required in comparison to few drops of essential oils. These oils are naturally present in the herbs and plants and not only is their individual effect of worth consideration.

Just like all other essential oils, frankincense oil has also got the ability of providing you with ultimate health benefits and it is also used widely as diffusers. This book is all about the best uses of frankincense essential oil diffusers and the ways by which you can use them during summers and winters.

Importance of essential oils as diffusers cannot be denied. So, you can use them without any difficulty and without any fear of side effects. In this book, I am going to tell you the importance of the natural essential oil diffusers along with some of the diffuser recipes which you should try in order to get your work done. If you are thinking that you may get any sort of side effects by using these oils then I must say, do not worry about the side effects at all.

Chapter 1 – An introduction to essential oil diffusers

Essential oils are very much beneficial for you if you use them for useful purposes. In the modern era when people prefer to use latest medicines and technology based treatments for getting better health, there are also present many herbal treatments as well which will help you out in getting rid of any problem you have. There are certain natural essential oils as well which can be matter if you are having any sort of skin problem or your hair are suffering from dryness, essential oils of every kind are avail which will assist you in getting flawless beauty and beautiful hair.

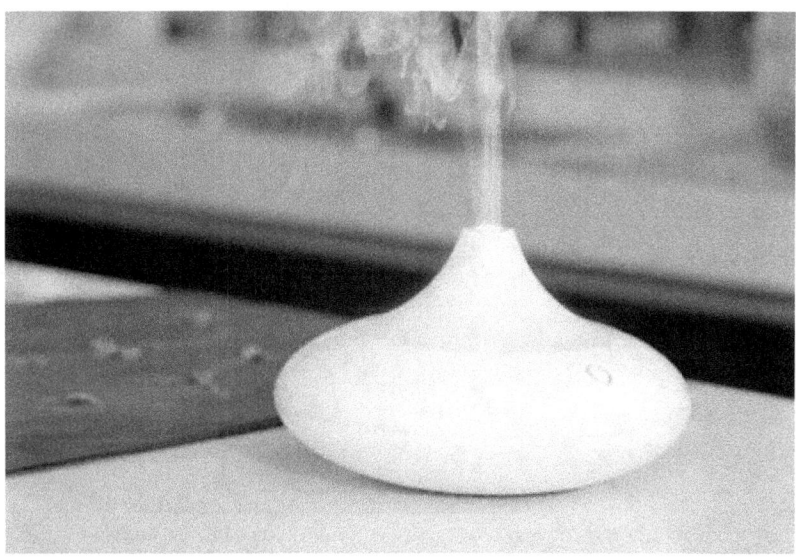

Just a little drop of natural oil at a time can bring calmness, can help us to focus on various things which are required, can help in reducing the tensions which we face. It can help in calming down our muscles, in making our digestion better and to make use physically and mentally strong to face the day to day challenges which come to our way.

Various combinations of essential oils in different kinds of recipes are also very much beneficial for the users. Just like all other essential oils, natural essential oil also helps you a lot in gaining extravagant benefits. There are so many uses of this essential oil and following are the main reasons why the natural oil is used in a variety of ways.

We are living a life where we are completely surrounded by numerous kinds of chemicals which are definitely not healthy for us and they are eventually making us sick. Like the detergents, soaps, air fresheners and numerous other things are there which are a part of our everyday life and are just adding negative impacts on our wellbeing.

While we are surrounded by so many unnatural harmful products, we are in need of using something which should grant us with unmatchable health benefits in a natural way. The essential oils prove to be so much beneficial in this regard. Without any doubt, essential oils are having ideal solutions in a natural way for the harmful effects.

It has been thousands of years for the essential oils are in use of humans and are providing ultimate and matchless benefits in many aspects. These oils have got therapeutic properties and are greatly used in the practice of aromatherapy as these oils are having some healing properties as well. The main source of essential oils is stems, leaves and roots of plants from where they are extracted.

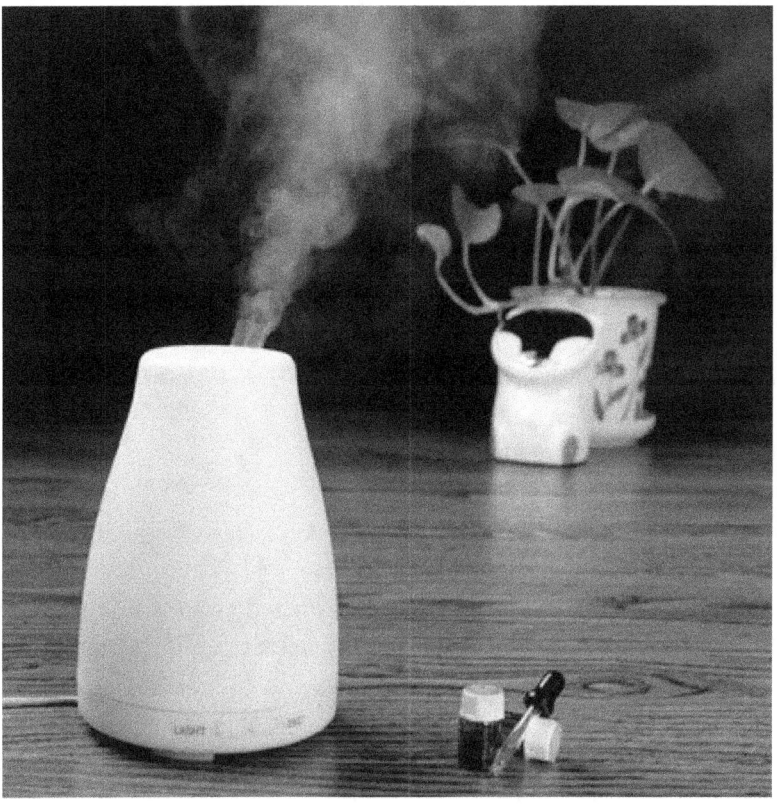

In the modern era, the lifestyle of people has seen a dramatic change. It can proved to be full of stress at many times but this stress can be taken away by one way or the other. In modern times, people are addicted to technology and the recent milestones which have been achieved by the scientists, but we cannot neglect this fact that the herbal and natural remedies which have been used by our ancestors cannot be overlooked at any cost.

These natural remedies from natural extracts have got so much power that they can make us feel better by one way or the other. It has been in practice since very long ago when generations after generations, people used to have the natural ingredients to make their life better. Despite of having so much latest medicines and technology in the modern era, the importance of those herbal extracts and their use in making the life better cannot be denied.

Today just like other things, the use of essential oils is also having so much significance and demand that no one can deny. In fact, these essential oils can be used not only for curing many kinds problems related to health but also helps in getting out of that problem without any side effects.

Since very long ago, the use of essential oils as a medicine and in many other aspects have been continued and they are actually very powerful natural agents which are being used for curing various types of problems and till present day the importance of these chemical free essential oils cannot be denied in any case. You can also use these oils as summer and spring diffusers with much ease.

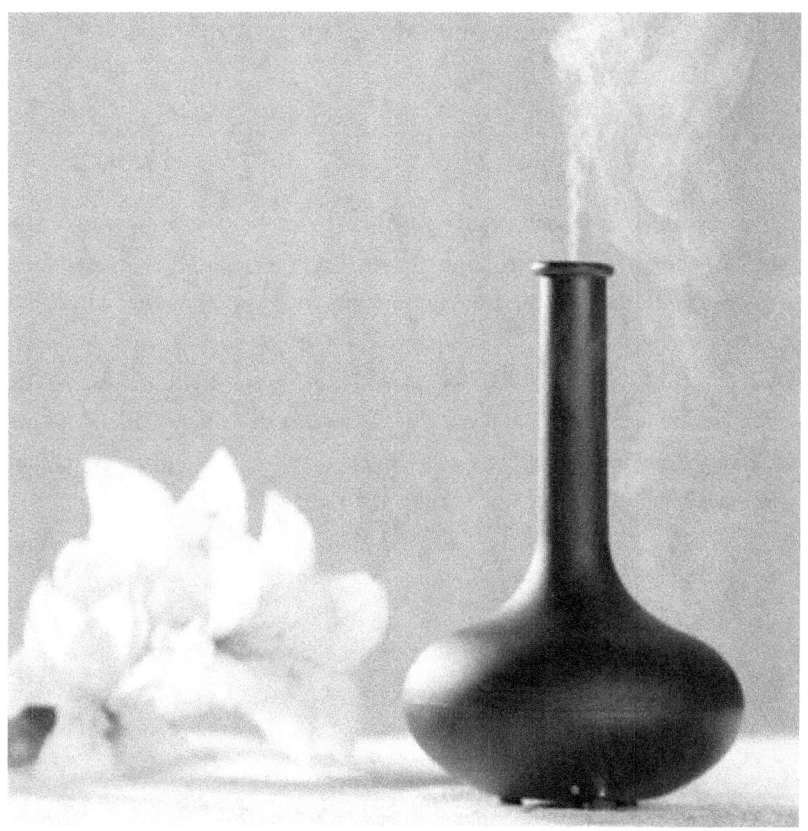

All of these essential oils are free of any chemicals which can proved to be harmful for your health. So, you can have use of all of these natural essential oil diffusers while keeping your eye even closed. In presence of so many modern techniques, essential oil's use cannot be deigned and if you want to get immense benefits out of it, you must use them as per the instructions as I am going to tell you. The main benefit of using these essential oils diffusers is that they can be used without any risk of getting any harm because they are free of any chemicals and harmful ingredients.

Chapter 2 – Why to opt for natural essential oil diffusers?

The herbs which are used for the extraction of essential oils are very much beneficial and are being in use for centuries. The oils are mostly extracted from the herbs and plants and are used for multiple purposes. The essential oils are extracted from various origins like orange peel, lemon peel, almond, lavender, eucalyptus etc. There is a much wider exposure of humans to these essential oils which are chemical free. The main benefit of using these essential oils for the treatment of anything is that these oils are completely deprived of any harmful or side effect thus you can use them in any way and for getting anything cured.

Exceptional properties

Not only this, but many of the essential oils have also got the property of having extra ordinary fragrance, so these oils can also be used as a fragrance and a very good example of such a fragrance is the rose essential oil, which is not only used for the tremens of various skin problems but also used as a fragrance and as an essential part of many concentrated perfumes.

Thus we can say that the essential oils have got immense importance which cannot be denied in any case and if you want to get all the bandits out of these oils you must follow all the steps and techniques of using the essential oils for treatment of any problem.

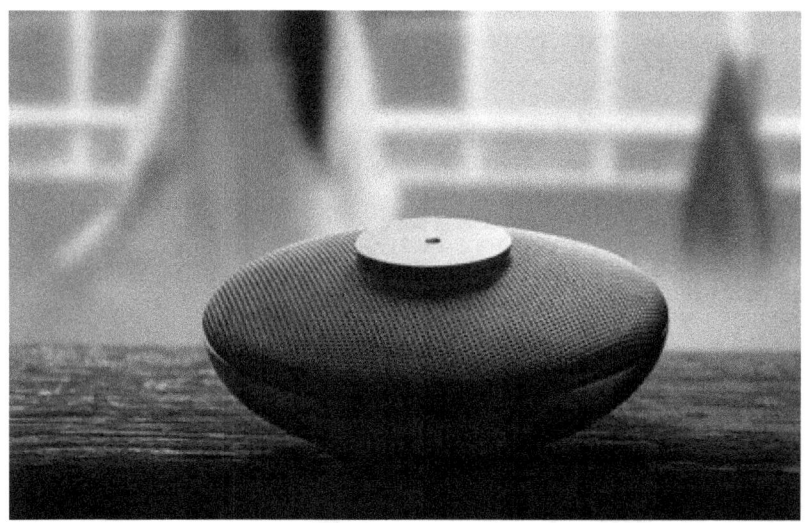

As far as the extent of choosing the right oils are concerned for making right fragrance, it is basically up to you that what kind of fragrance do you like and what are those ingredients which you want to be added as an essential component of deodorant you are making. Sometimes, you cannot become able to decide what to do with the ingredients you have. But do not worry at all as I have given the exact and perfect combination of different oils so that different types of fragrances can be made out of them.

The idea behind choosing the diffusers which I will be giving you in the coming chapters lies in the fact that I was thinking about different occasions where some kind of festivity or joy will be or different types of mood which I may have depending upon the environment in which I am present. So, you must be having the same thinking for sure as for different occasions you will be having different moods as well.

The diffusers which are manufactured synthetically can be composed of some harmful chemicals which can harm your skin and which should not be taken in to your consideration when you are looking for some diffuser in any local store near you. So, you are just in a need of having some organic essential oils so that you can use them without facing any problem.

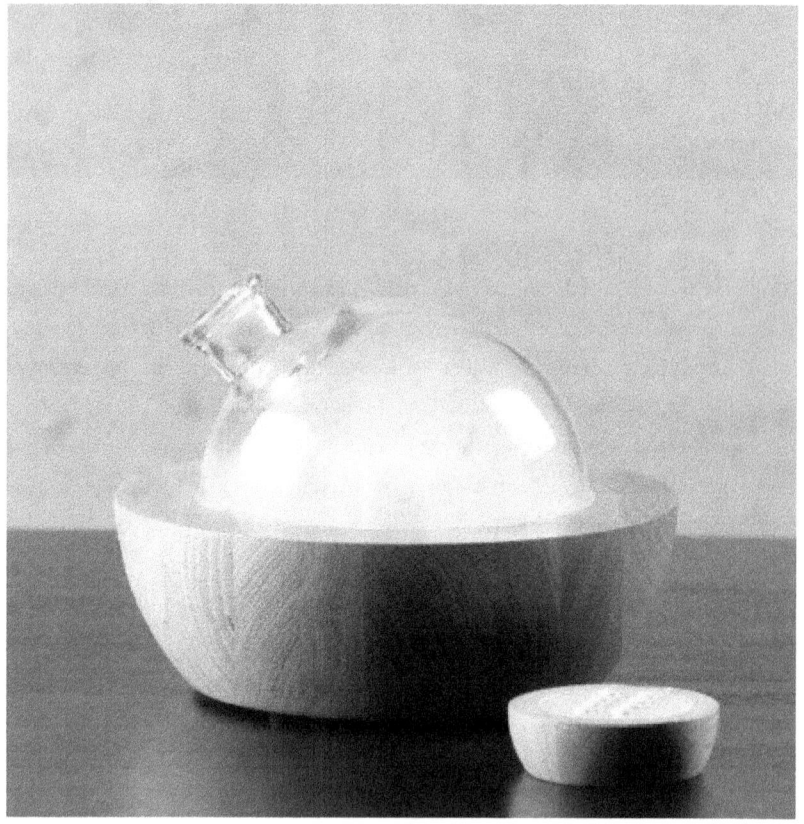

One important aspect of homemade diffuser is that, you can have their fragrance with you for quite a longer period of time, sometimes for all day, unlike that of synthetic diffusers who may disappear just after some time.

It is true that all of us having a desire of smelling something good which is good in fragrance and which is liked by everyone. If you get to have your own diffuser of your own then it will really be that thing full of fun for you when you will use it in routine at so many occasions and for so many reasons. This signature secret will make you able to have some unique value of yours as compared to the people who are around you as it is that smell that is exclusively being used by you and not by anyone else.

At this stage, you should not forget this in any case that when you are going to make your own diffuser with the help of organic ingredients, you should be patient enough to look for the right things to do. Do not do anything which can take you towards hurry and be there to exhibit patience as some diffuser require some days to get in to that consistency which you are desiring to have with you.

Chapter 3 – 20 essential oil diffuser recipes

Recipe no. 1

Ingredients:

- Jojoba oil three drops
- Almond oil four drops
- Jasmine essential oil four drops

Method:

- Take all the oils that have been mentioned in the detailed list of ingredients and their quantity above.
- Beware that you are taking the right quantity just according to what have been mentioned in the ingredients above.
- Leave the bottle for about four days in a dry place or you can also place it in the sun for four to four hours daily so that all the oils get mixed with each other with a high level of consistency.
- Then keep the bottle at a place with the lowest level of humidity.

Recipe no. 2

Ingredients:

- Honey three drops
- Jojoba oil three drops
- Carrot oil four drops
- Jasmine essential oil four drops
- Lemon oil three drops

Method:

- Take all the oils that have been mentioned in the detailed list of ingredients and their quantity above.
- Take a small bottle or container and add all the above-mentioned ingredients.
- Close the lid of the bottle and mix the oils very well.
- Leave the bottle for about four to three days so that all the oils get mixed with each other with a high level of consistency.
- Then keep the bottle in cool and dry place.
- Place the diffuser cap at the top of the bottle.

- Press the button to have its fumes out whenever you need.

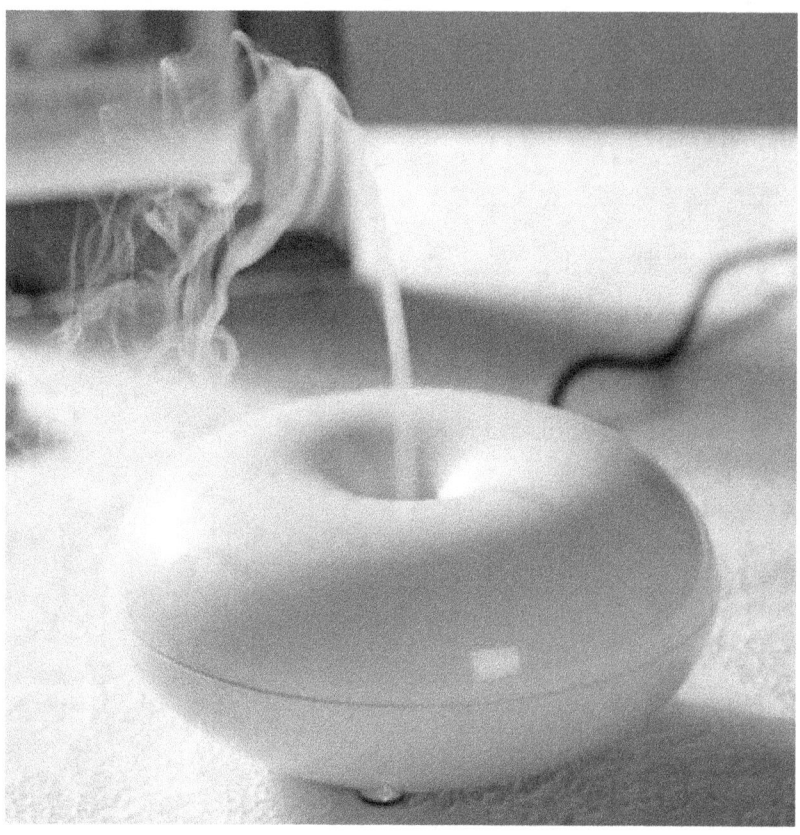

Recipe no. 3

Ingredients:

- Jojoba oil three drops
- Almond oil four drops
- Rose essential oil four drops
- Lemon oil four drops

Method:

- Take all the oils that have been mentioned in the detailed list of ingredients and their quantity above.
- Make the lid of the bottle closed and mix the oils well so that they can become smooth in consistency.
- Leave the bottle for about one day or 24 hours in a dry place or you can also place it in the sun for four to four hours daily so that all the oils get mixed with each other with a high level of consistency.
- Then keep the bottle at a place with the lowest level of humidity.
- Place the diffuser cap at the top of the bottle.
- Press the button to have its fumes out whenever you need.

Recipe no. 4

Ingredients:

- Lemon oil three drops
- Almond oil three drops
- Jojoba oil five drops
- Jasmine essential oil four drops

Method:

- Take all the oils that have been mentioned in the detailed list of ingredients and their quantity above.
- Take a small bottle or container and add all the ingredients that have been mentioned in the above-mentioned list for your convenience.
- Close the bottle's lid tightly so that no air can enter inside and mix all the mixtures well so that you can get the desired consistency out of it without any ambiguity on your way.
- Leave the bottle for about three to five days so that all the oils get mixed with each other with a high level of consistency.
- Place the diffuser cap at the top of the bottle.
- Press the button to have its fumes out whenever you need.

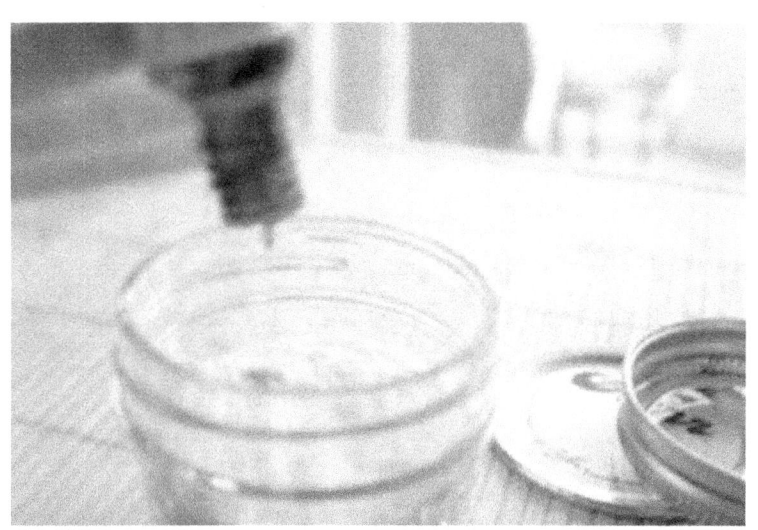

Recipe no. 5

Ingredients:

- Jojoba oil three drops
- Jasmine essential oil three drops
- Lemon oil four drops
- Almond oil four drops

Method:

- Take all the oils that have been mentioned in the detailed list of ingredients and their quantity above.
- Take a small bottle or container and add all the ingredients that have been mentioned in the above-mentioned list for your convenience.
- Make the lid of the bottle closed and mix the oils well so that they can become smooth in consistency.
- Now you should keep the bottle in dry place for about two to three days, so that all the ingredients get consistent.
- Place the diffuser cap at the top of the bottle.
- Press the button to have its fumes out whenever you need.

Recipe no. 6

Ingredients:

- Grapefruit oil three drops
- Jasmine essential oil four drops
- Sweet almond oil three drops
- Rose essential oil four drops

Method:

- Take all the oils that have been mentioned in the detailed list of ingredients and their quantity above.
- Beware that you are taking the right quantity just according to what have been mentioned in the ingredients above.
- Take a small bottle or container and add all the ingredients that have been mentioned in the above-mentioned list for your convenience.
- Leave the bottle for about four days in a dry place or you can also place it in the sun for four to four hours daily so that all the oils get mixed with each other with a high level of consistency.
- Place the diffuser cap at the top of the bottle.
- Press the button to have its fumes out whenever you need.

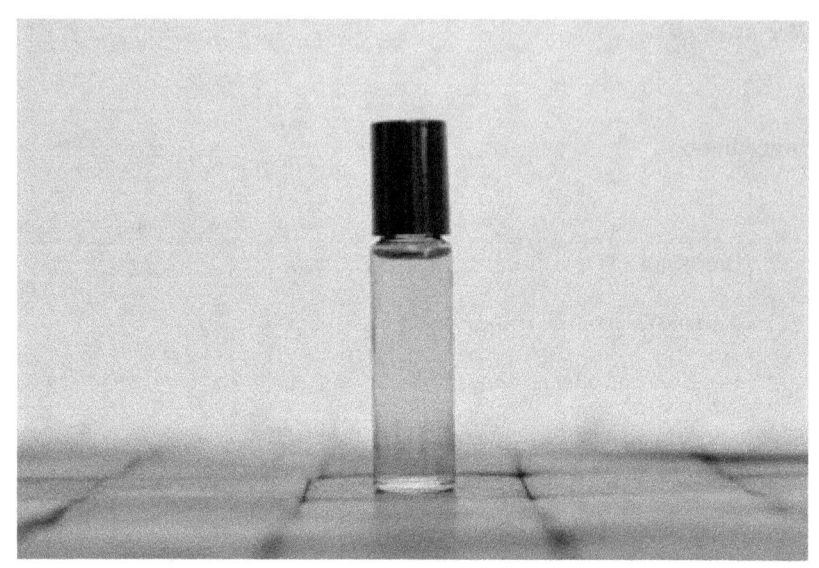

Recipe no. 7

Ingredients:

- Almond oil three drops
- Almond oil three drops
- Jasmine oil four drops
- Jasmine essential oil four drops

Method:

- Take all the oils that have been mentioned in the detailed list of ingredients.
- Beware that you are taking the right quantity as it is mentioned above.
- Take a small bottle or container and add all the ingredients that have been mentioned in the above-mentioned list for your convenience.
- Place the diffuser cap at the top of the bottle.
- Press the button to have its fumes out, whenever you need.

Recipe no. 8

Ingredients:

- Nutmeg oil three drops
- Rosemary oil four drops
- Jasmine essential oil four drops
- Almond oil four drops
- Black cumin oil four drops

Method:

- Take all the oils that have been above.
- Close the bottle's lid tightly so that no air can enter inside and mix all the mixtures well so that you can get the desired consistency out of it without any ambiguity on your way.
- Now you should keep the bottle in dry place for about two to three days, so that all the ingredients get consistent.
- Then keep the bottle in cool place.
- Place the diffuser cap at the top of the bottle.
- Press the button to have its fumes out whenever you need.
- Apply it to neck, back of year and wrist to get elegant fragrance.

Recipe no. 9

Ingredients:

- Lavender oil four drops
- Almond oil three drops
- Jojoba oil four drops
- Lemon oil three drops

Method:

- Take all the ingredients mentioned above in a small bottle with a cap.
- Beware that you are taking the right quantity just according to what have been mentioned in the ingredients above.
- Take a small bottle or container and add all the ingredients that have been mentioned in the above-mentioned list for your convenience.
- Now you should keep the bottle in dry place for about two to three days, so that all the ingredients get consistent.
- Place the diffuser cap at the top of the bottle.
- Press the button to have its fumes out whenever you need.
- Apply it to neck, back of year and wrist to get elegant fragrance.

Recipe no. 10

Ingredients:

- Almond oil three drops
- Cilantro oil four drops
- Jasmine essential oil 2 drops

Method:

- Take all the ingredients mentioned above in a small bottle with a cap.
- Beware that you are taking the right quantity as it is mentioned above.
- Close the bottle's lid tightly so that no air can enter inside and mix all the mixtures well.
- Place the diffuser cap at the top of the bottle.
- Press the button to have its fumes out whenever you need.
- Apply the body spray at the back of the ear, in front of neck, on the chest or at any place of your body where you are having the desire to apply it.

Recipe no. 11

Ingredients:

- Almond oil 3 teaspoon
- Lemon juice 3 drops
- Jasmine essential oil 3 drops
- Lemon oil 3 drops

Method:

- Take a small container and add all the ingredients that have been mentioned above.
- Close the cap of the container and mix the oils well.
- Leave the container for about 3 days so that the body spray can be enriched.
- Place the diffuser cap at the top of the bottle.
- Press the button to have its fumes out whenever you need.
- Apply the body spray at the back of the ear, in front of neck, or at any place of your body where you want.

Recipe no. 12

Ingredients:

- Rosemary oil 3 drops
- Almond oil 3 drops
- Raspberry essential oil 3 drops
- Jasmine essential oil 9 drops

Method:

- Take a small container and add all the ingredients that have been mentioned above.
- Make the cap of the bottle closed and mix the oils well so that they can become smooth in consistency.
- Leave the bottle for about 5 days in a dry place or you can also place it in the sun for 3 to 3 hours daily so that the body spray can be enriched.
- Then keep the bottle at a place with the lowest level of humidity.
- Place the diffuser cap at the top of the bottle.
- Press the button to have its fumes out whenever you need.

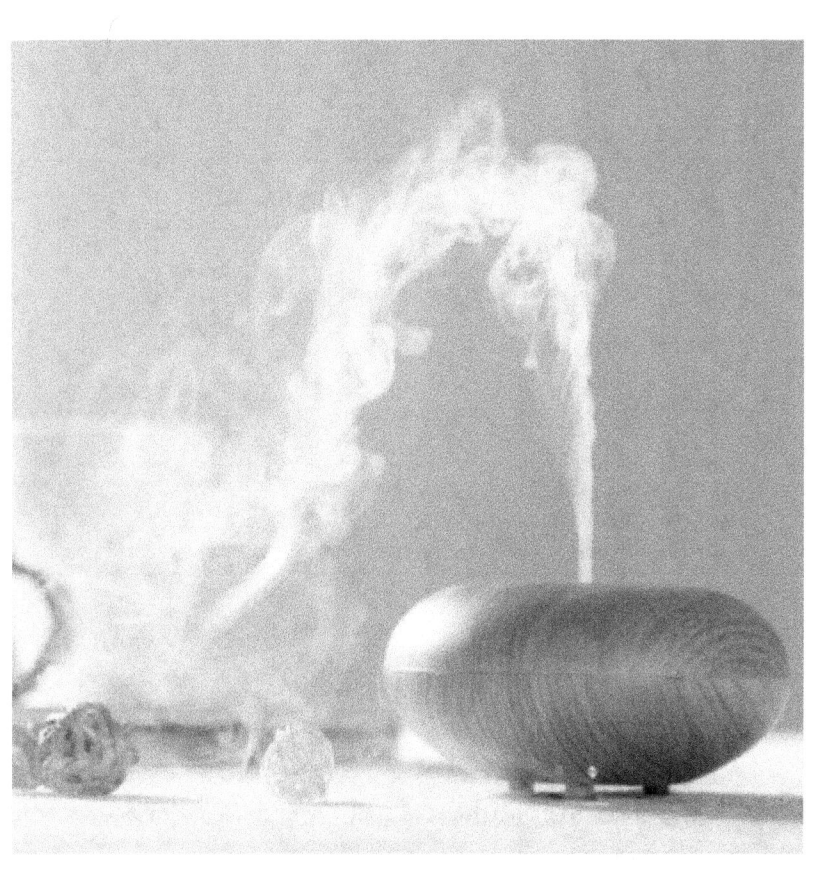

Recipe no. 13

Ingredients:

- Cumin oil 3 drops
- Ginger oil 3 drops
- Grapefruit oil 3 drops
- Jasmine essential oil 3 drops
- Raspberry essential oil 3 drops

Method:

- Take a small container and add all the ingredients that have been mentioned above.
- Close the bottle's cap tightly so that no air can enter inside and mix all the mixtures well so that you can get the desired consistency out of it without any ambiguity on your way.
- Leave the bottle for about 3 days so that the body spray can be enriched.
- Then keep the bottle in cool and dry place.
- Place the diffuser cap at the top of the bottle.
- Press the button to have its fumes out whenever you need.

Recipe no. 14

Ingredients:

- Rosemary oil 3 drops
- Almond oil 3 drops
- Raspberry essential oil 3 drops
- Jasmine essential oil 3 drops

Method:

- Take all the oils that have been mentioned in the detailed list of ingredients and their quantity above.
- Beware that you are taking the right quantity as it is mentioned above.
- Close the bottle's cap tightly so that no air can enter inside.
- Mix all the mixtures well so that you can get the desired consistency out of it.
- Then keep the bottle in cool and dry place.
- Place the diffuser cap at the top of the bottle.
- Press the button to have its fumes out whenever you need.

Recipe no. 15

Ingredients:

- Almond oil 3 drops
- Cilantro oil 3 drops
- Jasmine essential oil 3 drops
- Raspberry essential oil 3 drops
- Cumin oil 3 drops

Method:

- Take a small bottle or container and add all the ingredients that have been mentioned in the above-mentioned list for your convenience.
- Make the cap of the bottle closed and mix the oils well so that they can become smooth in consistency.
- Leave the bottle for about 3 days in a dry place or you can also place it in the sun for 3 to 3 hours daily so that the body spray can be enriched.
- Then keep the bottle at a place with the lowest level of humidity. Place the diffuser cap at the top of the bottle.
- Press the button to have its fumes out whenever you need.

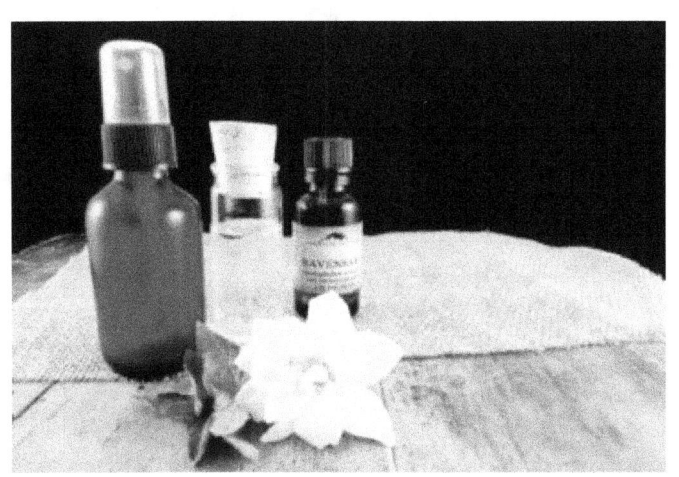

Recipe no. 16

Ingredients:

- Rose essential oil 3 drops
- Jasmine essential oil 3 drops
- Cumin oil 3 drops
- Lemon oil 3 drops
- Savory oil 3 drops

Method:

- Take a small bottle or container and add all the ingredients that have been mentioned in the above-mentioned list for your convenience.
- Close the bottle's cap tightly so that no air can enter inside and mix all the mixtures well so that you can get the desired consistency out of it without any ambiguity on your way.
- Then keep the bottle in cool and dry place.
- Place the diffuser cap at the top of the bottle.
- Press the button to have its fumes out whenever you need.

Recipe no. 17

Ingredients:

- Almond essential oil 3 teaspoon
- Turmeric oil 3 drops
- Clementine oil 3 drops
- Clove bud oil 3 drops

Method:

- Take a small bottle or container and add all the ingredients that have been mentioned in the above-mentioned list for your convenience.
- Make the cap of the bottle closed and mix the oils well so that they can become smooth in consistency.
- Leave the bottle for about 3 days in a dry place or you can also place it in the sun for 3 to 3 hours daily so that the body spray can be enriched.
- Then keep the bottle at a place with the lowest level of humidity.
- Place the diffuser cap at the top of the bottle.
- Press the button to have its fumes out whenever you need.

Recipe no. 18

Ingredients:

- Rose essential oil 3 drops
- Rosemary essential oil 3 teaspoon
- Jasmine essential oil 3 teaspoon
- Apple cider vinegar half cup

Method:

- Take a small bottle or container and add all the ingredients that have been mentioned in the above-mentioned list for your convenience.
- Close the bottle's cap tightly so that no air can enter inside and mix all the mixtures well so that you can get the desired consistency out of it without any ambiguity on your way.
- Place the diffuser cap at the top of the bottle.
- Press the button to have its fumes out whenever you need.

Recipe no. 19

Ingredients:

- Coconut oil 3 teaspoon
- Rosemary essential oil 3 teaspoon
- Lemongrass oil 3 teaspoon
- Cumin oil 3 drops
- Vanilla oil 3 drops
- Sage oil 3 drops

Method:

- Take all the oils and ingredients.
- Take a small bottle or container and add all the ingredients that have been mentioned in the above-mentioned list for your convenience.
- Close the cap of the bottle and mix the oils well.
- Then keep the bottle in cool and dry place.
- Place the diffuser cap at the top of the bottle.
- Press the button to have its fumes out whenever you need.

Recipe no. 20

Ingredients:

- Rosemary oil 2 teaspoon
- Coconut oil 3 teaspoon
- Grapefruit oil 4 drops
- Celery seed oil 4 drops
- Black pepper oil 2 drops

Method:

- Take a small container and add all the ingredients that have been mentioned above.
- Beware that you are taking the right quantity just according to what have been mentioned in the ingredients above.
- Make the cap of the bottle closed and mix the oils well so that they can become smooth in consistency.
- Leave the bottle for about 3 days in a dry place or you can also place it in the sun for 3 to 3 hours daily so that the body spray can be enriched.
- Place the diffuser cap at the top of the bottle.
- Press the button to have its fumes out whenever you need.

Chapter 4 – 10 spring and summer essential oil diffuser recipes

Recipe no. 1

Ingredients:

Jojoba oil 4 drops

Almond oil 4 drops

Poppy seeds 2 teaspoon

Method:

- Mix all ingredients.
- Leave in dry place for about two days.
- Place the diffuser cap at the top of the bottle.
- Press the button to have its fumes out whenever you need.

Recipe no. 2

Ingredients:

Honey 4 drops

Jojoba oil 4 drops

Carrot oil 4 drops

Orange peel essential oil 2 drops

Method:

- Combine all ingredients.
- Leave in dry place for about two days.
- Place the diffuser cap at the top of the bottle.
- Press the button to have its fumes out whenever you need.

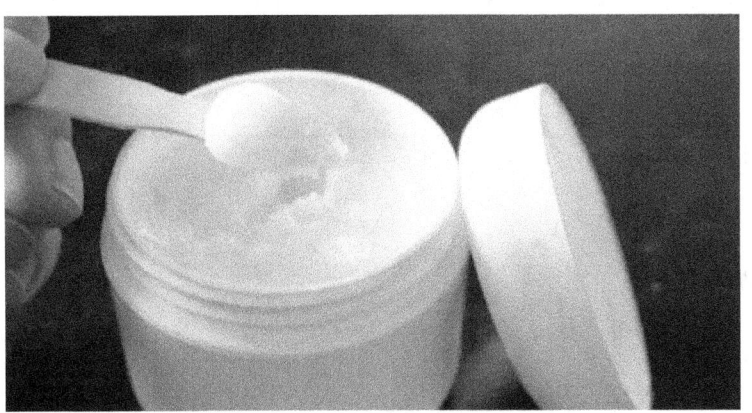

Recipe no. 3

Ingredients:

Jojoba oil 4 drops

Turmeric powder 1 teaspoon

Hazel drops 1 teaspoon

Method:

- Combine all ingredients.
- Then keep the bottle in cool and dry place.
- Place the diffuser cap at the top of the bottle.
- Press the button to have its fumes out whenever you need.

Recipe no. 4

Ingredients:

Lemon essential oil 4 drops

Almond oil 2 drops

Strawberry essential oil 2 drops

Method:

- Combine all ingredients.
- Then keep the bottle in cool and dry place.
- Place the diffuser cap at the top of the bottle.
- Press the button to have its fumes out whenever you need.

Recipe no. 5

Ingredients:

- Rose essential oil 3 drops
- Lemon oil 3 drops

Method:

- Take a small bottle or container and add all the ingredients that have been mentioned in the above-mentioned list for your convenience.
- Then keep the bottle in cool and dry place.
- Place the diffuser cap at the top of the bottle.
- Press the button to have its fumes out whenever you need.

Recipe no. 6

Ingredients:

Tea tree oil 2 teaspoon

Peppermint oil 1 teaspoon

Almond oil 4 drops

Method:

- Combine all ingredients.
- Then keep the bottle in cool and dry place.
- Place the diffuser cap at the top of the bottle.
- Press the button to have its fumes out whenever you need.

Recipe no. 7

Ingredients:

- Rose essential oil 3 drops
- Jasmine essential oil 3 drops
- Cumin oil 3 drops
- Lemon oil 3 drops
- Savory oil 3 drops

Method:

- Take a small bottle or container and add all the ingredients that have been mentioned in the above-mentioned list for your convenience.
- Close the bottle's cap tightly so that no air can enter inside and mix all the mixtures well so that you can get the desired consistency out of it without any ambiguity on your way.
- Then keep the bottle in cool and dry place.
- Place the diffuser cap at the top of the bottle.
- Press the button to have its fumes out whenever you need.

Recipe no. 8

Ingredients:

Jojoba oil 4 drops

Raspberry oil 2 teaspoon

Method:

- Combine all ingredients.
- Then keep the bottle in cool and dry place.
- Place the diffuser cap at the top of the bottle.
- Press the button to have its fumes out whenever you need.

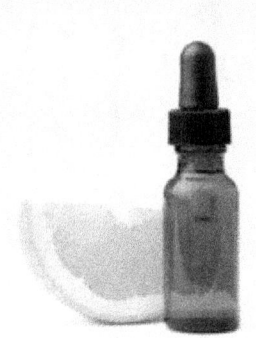

Recipe no. 9

Ingredients:

- Rose essential oil 3 drops
- Jasmine essential oil 3 drops
- Cumin oil 3 drops
- Lemon oil 3 drops
- Savory oil 3 drops

Method:

- Take a small bottle or container and add all the ingredients above.
- Close the bottle's cap tightly so that no air can enter inside and mix all the mixtures well so that you can get the desired consistency out of it without any ambiguity on your way.
- Then keep the bottle in cool and dry place.
- Place the diffuser cap at the top of the bottle.
- Press the button to have its fumes out whenever you need.

Recipe no. 10

Ingredients:

Jojoba oil 3 drops

Hazel 1 teaspoon

Almond oil 4 drops

Raspberry essential oil

Method:

- Combine all ingredients.
- Then keep the bottle in cool and dry place.
- Place the diffuser cap at the top of the bottle.
- Press the button to have its fumes out whenever you need.

Conclusion

The essential oils have got so many exceptional properties which can distinguish them from many other treatments as well. They sometimes act as anti-bacterial, anti-viral and antiseptic properties which are really helpful in getting out of all those problems which are caused by bacteria, virus or any other microbes.

Essential oils can grant you so many benefits which you cannot even imagine form any other source. Although, the modern people consider the use of modern medicines for curing many kinds of health problems but the use of essential oils is by far considered more effective and efficient as compared to any other thing. They can be used as summer diffusers and you will then not need to buy any deodorant from market again without any problem.

FREE Bonus Reminder

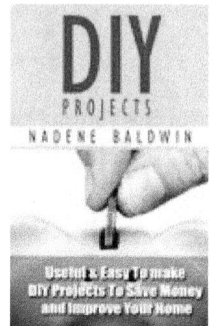

If you have not grabbed it yet, please go ahead and download your special bonus report *"DIY Projects. 13 Useful & Easy To Make DIY Projects To Save Money & Improve Your Home!"*

Simply Click the Button Below

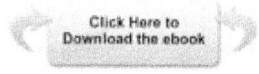

OR **Go to This Page**

http://diyhomecraft.com/free

BONUS #2: More Free & Discounted Books

Do you want to receive more Free & Discounted Books?

We have a mailing list where we send out our new Books when they go free or with a discount on Kindle. Click on the link below to sign up for Free & Discount Book Promotions.

=> Sign Up for Free & Discount Book Promotions <=

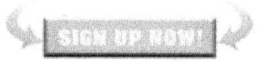

OR Go to this URL

http://zbit.ly/1WBb1Ek

www.ingramcontent.com/pod-product-compliance
Lightning Source LLC
Chambersburg PA
CBHW071132280526
45787CB00003B/1259